WHEN
YOUR CHILD
IS OVERWEIGHT

WHEN YOUR CHILD IS OVERWEIGHT

Leslie-Jane Maynard

ABBEY PRESS

St. Meinrad, Indiana 47577

To Craig and Elizabeth Ann

ACKNOWLEDGEMENT

I thank Susan Wisner Rushmore for contributing her creativity, intelligence, and technical assistance to the development of this manuscript.

Without her total dedication, this project would not have been possible.

PHOTO CREDITS: Deborah Churan, Cover; Bob Taylor, pages 8 and 44-45; Paul Conklin, pages 25 and 79; Berne Greene, page 62.

Library of Congress Catalog Card Number
79-55863
ISBN: 0-87029-162-9

CONTENTS

Preface

This book has been written for parents of overweight children. Along with giving practical advice, I feel it important to offer insights into the emotional obstacles encountered by the overweight child and parent. A parent can be justifiably frustrated, bewildered, or angered by an emotionally taxing child with a weight problem. This is especially true since such a child is likely to also be frustrated, bewildered, and angry.

A youngster's overweight problem is not the child's alone; it involves the entire family. Both parent and child are hurting. This book attempts to help parent and child communicate in a constructive manner. I want to help both parties learn to work together and to assist them in establishing a constructive and loving relationship. I am concerned with health: the health of the relationships within the family, the health of the child's body, and his or her emotional well-being.

For my knowledge in this area, I am indebted to every overweight child I have ever worked with. Each one helped me to understand his or her needs. I am equally grateful to the parents of these overweight children. As they shared their most pressing problems, I became aware of what they needed most to solve their difficulties. May what I share in this book ease your burden, and that of your child.

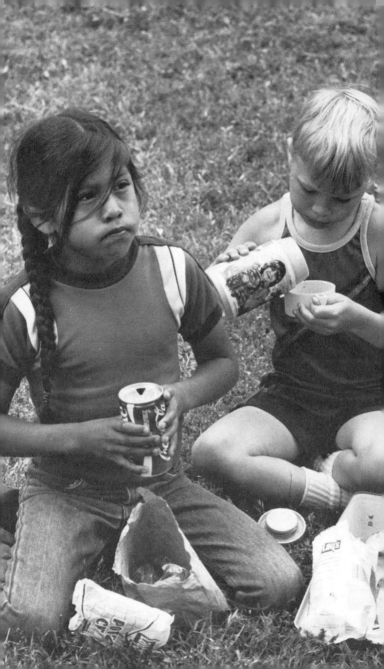

CHAPTER 1

The Overweight Child

"I prepare a slimming breakfast, lunch, and dinner for my ten-year-old Lisa, and yet she seems to get heavier every day. I don't know what to do. I have tried talking to our pediatrician, but all she says is, 'She has a hearty appetite and will outgrow it.'

"Sometimes Lisa comes home from school saying that the other children call her bad names. My heart breaks for her, and I just want to hold her. I tell her that the reason the other children talk that way is that they are cruel. Deep in my heart, I know exactly what Lisa is going through. I was once an overweight little girl myself.

"The other day, when Lisa's teacher called, I was mortified. She had noticed that Lisa was trading her carrot sticks and celery for cookies and cupcakes. She wondered if I was aware of the problem.

"Of late, Lisa no longer plays with the other children when she comes home from school. She just sits in front of the television and looks sad. When I suggest to her that she put on her play clothes, her only comment is: 'Mommy, I am too tired.'

"Taking Lisa shopping for clothes is a nightmare. She points to all the cute little dresses she cannot possibly fit into. The dressing room becomes a scene of tears and heartbreak. Lisa must buy her clothes in the chubby department, but she refuses to acknowledge this.

"Sometimes, I am so frustrated that I just let Lisa do whatever she wants to with food. I could hardly believe it the other day when she ate a whole box of cookies.

"My husband and I went to Open School Week. Lisa's teacher reported that her academic progress is adequate, but she was concerned because Lisa never joins in any of the children's games. She was also worried because Lisa does not socialize, and she verified that the other children in the class are not kind to her.

"From the classroom we went to see Lisa's gym teacher, who told us that Lisa seldom participates in any of the activities. The teacher felt that, because Lisa is so overweight, it is physically difficult for her to do cartwheels, play tag, and climb the rope. She said that Lisa spends most of her time in gym class sitting in a corner with her head buried in her lap.

"We then went to visit with Lisa's music

teacher. We were told that Lisa has an exceptionally sweet voice and is very musical. We were elated to get some positive comments on our daughter, but our elation was soon over when we spoke to the school nurse.

"The nurse informed us that Lisa is 14 pounds above the normal weight for girls of her age. We were admonished for not looking after Lisa's weight problem. Did we realize that Lisa was heading for possible physical, emotional, and psychological problems?"

From her mother's account, it is clear that Lisa's life today is not pleasant. The child knows only that she has a ravenous appetite, few friends, poor experiences with other children in school, and very frustrated parents.

Being different from the peer group may lead to emotionally unbearable feelings of inadequacy in the overweight child. The youngster may try to overcome these feelings by eating more, which only exacerbates those emotions which led to the eating in the first place. The overweight child must unlearn the link between emotional discomfort and finding solace in food, but is not yet mature enough to do so. The parent is usually bewildered, searching for answers. Many times the school only records the child's behavior problems and/or lack of academic progress, and turns the problem back to the parents.

Too often the overweight child does not receive from parents the emotional or practical support, love, and understanding that a child with an obvious physical impairment elicits. Reactions to a child's obesity are more likely to be shame and anger. This stems not from any lack of parental love, but rather from simply not understanding the complexity of the problem of obesity. This misunderstanding engenders many negative feelings in both parent and child.

Understanding can begin with an awareness of the causes of obesity which are either endogenous or exogenous. Endogenous obesity ("endo" meaning "inside") results from genetic (inherited), hypothalamic (glandular), and metabolic (the rate at which the body burns fuel) causes. This means that the child's weight problem results from a physical malfunctioning which can be diagnosed and treated medically.

Exogenous ("exo" meaning "outside") obesity results from cultural, emotional, environmental, behavioral, and/or economic causes. The body is healthy, but outside forces are influencing weight. This type of obesity is by far the most common, affecting about 90% of overweight children. Nearly one-third of all Americans are obese. This means 60 to 70 million people in this country are overweight.

Let us explore, one by one, the causes of exogenous, or nonmedical, obesity in children.

1. **Cultural:** A child may be overweight simply because it is thought by the family that a chubby child is a healthy, well-adjusted one. If you have old family albums, are the people in them somewhat overweight? Your mother?

Your grandfather? If so, it might well have been an accepted family pattern, almost an expectation, that children be chubby. This can help you understand why your own child might be overweight today.

To illustrate cultural influence on eating patterns and weight problems, let us look at a study contrasting American and French children. This study tells of a month-long cross-cultural obesity survey done by a medical student at a French university.

The findings reveal that only "perhaps one-half of one percent" of the 700 French children studied (ages 1-6) were overweight. In stark contrast to this, 737 New York children in the same age group had "an obesity prevalence of 10-20 percent." Obesity in the study was defined as a weight of 120% "the normal weight as shown on weight/height charts." The researcher uncovered some interesting cultural patterns in France that contribute to French children being less obese: sandwiches are thinner, meals are smaller, desserts are uncommon, and French children "have access to considerably less junk food . . . food served in a typical French home is not as rich as the food Americans are used to being served in French restaurants in the U.S."

While there well may be a genetic factor that could, in part at least, account for these findings, we can discern distinct differences in the attitudes of the French and Americans toward food. If you were to visit a French supermarket, you would find the packages to be much smaller. Our yogurt comes in pint containers, we have giant-sized boxes of cereal and family-sized packages of almost everything. The bigger, the better; quantity has taken the place of quality. We are told by the advertising people that if it's new and if it's large, it's good. Perhaps the obesity problem in this country is so widespread because of this bigger-is-better attitude.

The French seem to give more thought and attention to the appearance and quality of the food they serve. Mass production of food is more common in the United States. We seem to prefer to heat up something which has been mass produced, rather than take the time to prepare an item at home which, although smaller, could be quite special.

Is part of your child's weight problem the fact that portions you serve at meals are too large? You are not alone in this. You may be trapped by the prevailing national attitude. The next time you are in a grocery store, take a moment and look at the advertisement for the free cookbook on the carton of Old Fashioned Quaker Oats. This ad tells us several things about the attitude towards food in our culture. First, the book is free. Of course. That way, we will be sure to buy more oats. Second, and most alarming but quite to the point, is the phrase printed across the bottom of the ad. In bold letters stands the sentence: "The more they eat the better you feel."

14

Try to be honest with yourself. Have you unwittingly programmed your child to want more and more food, to expect large servings in place of fine-quality food? Have you given any thought to the visual appearance of your meals? To texture? These are elements of the eating experience which, by and large, Americans neglect.

2. Emotional: For the overweight child, eating may be an outlet for emotional strain that other children handle differently. Some children, for example, bite their nails; others may develop insomnia; still others may behave disruptively or react to emotional stress by stuttering. In all such cases, the task is to enable the child to handle feelings in positive, constructive ways.

3. Environmental: Surroundings may be playing a great role if a child is overeating. Is food available to the child at all times of the day? Are there filled candy dishes around the house? Have you watched children's Saturday morning television programming and noticed the advertising? The media are forever trying to get us to buy food, and you will find that the ads directed to children are usually for empty starches and sugars, unnutritious but weight producing. You must realize that your child is under tremendous pressure from this public onslaught, and to help solve the weight problem, you must try to re-educate your child's tastes as well as eating habits.

4. Behavioral: A child may overeat

15

simply out of habit. Your child may follow a routine of having a snack after school. There are other such simple behavioral patterns or habits: ice cream with television, popcorn in the movies, hotdogs at ball games, the bedtime milk and cookies.

5. **Economic:** Weight problems may begin simply because there is not enough money available for high-quality foods. The parent may turn to low-cost, high-starch items in order to stretch the budget, not knowing which protein foods are inexpensive. The children are thus encouraged to satisfy their hunger with carbohydrates. This is not to say that weight problems are limited to those with inadequate incomes. The opposite problem may exist: there may be an overavailability of money for food resulting in too much food being put before the child.

It is helpful for parents to list what they consider to be some of the causes of their child's weight problem. A child's obesity is an issue parents must come to grips with. This can only be done if the mother and father know the facts and are willing to deal with them. Chapter Two examines some truths and myths that surround the issue of the overweight child.

CHAPTER 2

Truths and Myths about Obesity

Your child has inherited your genes, your body structure, your features. Perhaps also your predisposition towards obesity, should you have such. He or she is also likely to adopt many of your behavior traits. Let us look at some statistics which bear out the influence of heredity on childhood obesity.

A study involving 189 obese children produced several interesting findings:

1. The children were at least 20% above the ideal weights for their ages.

2. Based on adult life insurance weight tables, it was revealed that, as a group, the parents of these children were significantly obese. Of the 189 women, 55 weighed over 175 pounds and 67 of the 189 men were over 200 pounds.

3. There is a correlation between obesity and some illnesses in children. Five of the

children had high blood pressure, which disappeared with weight correction.

4. The data indicates that children are equally responsive to programs for weight reduction whether or not their parents are obese.

The statistics from this study correlate with the findings of another recent medical survey. Both prove that there is indeed a strong hereditary factor in obesity: the weights of natural children correlate with those of their parents, while the weights of adopted children show no relationship to those of their foster parents. Of the obese children, 60 to 88% have one or both parents who are overweight.

Childhood obesity persists into adult life. After 20 years, 86% of obese boys and 80% of obese girls remained overweight. In contrast, only 42% of nonobese boys and 18% of nonobese girls were overweight 20 years later. I believe, more than ever, that if we could successfully treat every case of childhood obesity, we could prevent adult obesity.

Heredity and behavior-patterning are important influences in the development of childhood obesity. Equally contributing to the problem can be the myths about obesity. Consider the following true/false statements:

1. Some children can eat more than others without gaining weight.

True. Metabolic rates vary among children as they do with adults. Each individual human body is a finely tuned instrument, different from all the others.

2. Some children have an inborn liking for sweets.

False. A taste for sweets is acquired, not inherited.

3. The structure of some children's bodies will make them appear heavy.

True. Skeletal structure is inherited, not developed. Body type is inborn, and there are three distinct body types: the ectomorphic, the endomorphic, and the mesomorphic. The mesomorphic individual will tend to look heavier, as the basic build is stocky and truncated. The covering of the bony structure—flesh, fat and muscle—is determined by nutrition and exercise.

4. Sugar is higher in calories than honey.

False. Tablespoon for tablespoon, honey is higher: 61 calories per tablespoon versus 48.

5. Weight will be gained if food is eaten just before bedtime.

Generally false. The principle of "a calorie is a calorie" stands. The energy provided by calories is burned over a period of 24 hours. As long as the energy expended is equal to the caloric intake, there will be no weight gain. There are some studies indicating that laboratory animals lose at a faster rate merely by altering their feeding schedules, but the difference is insignificant. What is really important is the total caloric consumption.

6. Consuming an excessive amount of fluids will put on weight.

False. Calorie-free beverages do not add fat. There will be a temporary weight gain due to fluid retention. This water-weight will disappear if there is no medical complication. Ingestion of too much salt will retain water.

7. Protein calories are burned faster than carbohydrate calories.

False. A calorie is a calorie, no matter what the source. One pound is added by 3,500 calories. You will gain this pound whether you overeat on sugar or on cottage cheese.

8. Exercise must be part of a weight-loss program in order for it to succeed.

False. Although physical activity is desirable, it is not absolutely essential. Many overweight children who were immobilized, many confined to wheelchairs, have been successful.

9. The compulsive eater is addicted to food.

False. Overeating is a compulsion, and nothing more. If you have an obese child, you can understand the problem by thinking of something you do compulsively. Must you wash dishes immediately after eating? Do you smoke compulsively? Are you a compulsive worker? There are many funny little quirks in all of us, from having to read the newspaper every day, starting with the sports section and going backwards, to returning to the house ten times to be sure the stove is off. Overeating can be just another compulsion.

Overeating has been likened to alcoholism and drug addiction. I do not believe this to be valid. Alcohol and drugs are truly addictive substances. It is impossible to be addicted to pound cake and gumdrops. A person can, however, believe that he or she has no control over food. The body is governed by the mind.

Sugar itself is an exception. Especially in hypoglycemics and diabetics, true physiological sugar cravings do occur. For a normal person who is used to ingesting a certain amount of sugar, there may be a withdrawal period, just as there is when one gives up coffee or cigarettes.

Unless there is an organic cause, in my opinion, overeating is not a physical disease. There are many causes of obesity in children and adolescents. Some children are assumed to overeat because of "oral needs," some may eat in response to stressful situations. Boredom and the way food is advertised have also been suggested as contributing factors.

In infancy, overfeeding may take place because of the emotional needs of mothers or because of pressure from well-meaning husbands, grandmothers, or other relatives, or friends. Many times, adults will take pride in the fact that their child is such a "good eater," or "has such a healthy appetite." Overfeeding can also occur because of the parent's ignorance about correct weights for infants and children or lack of knowledge about what food intake is appropriate.

It is true that your child is much more apt to be overweight if you, yourself, are obese. Since you have undertaken the responsibility of

21

parenthood, this might be a good time for you to evaluate your own weight, especially if you have a problem with it, for this is likely to have an effect on your child.

CHAPTER 3
The Teenager's Plight

The teenage years are most often turbulent times for both parent and child. These times are troubled enough for every adolescent; compounded by a weight problem, life can seem even more difficult. The youngster who is going through the normal trials of maturing but who is hampered by weight may have a disastrous teenagehood.

As parents, we might think of the teen years as carefree ones, without the responsibilities of adulthood. This is, of course, what we would wish for our children. For ourselves, we would like to be granted some peace as our children grow. We have been through diaper changing, playground babysitting, the first day of school, clipping on mittens to coat sleeves, measles, mumps, Little League, Girl Scouts, sewing on name tapes for camp, etc. We are ready for our child to be more independent. We hope it's time to relax.

To the contrary. We must now change our ways of dealing with our children. There will be less physical interaction; this will be replaced by considerably more emotional interplay. Given the rebellious nature of most adolescents, it is highly unlikely that your teenager will want to take counsel from you about a weight problem. This is true especially if you give advice in a condescending manner. The adolescent is just beginning to feel him- or herself a person, and wants to be treated like an adult, even though adolescent behavior is very often still childlike.

You will probably have less control over your adolescent. Many more meals, for example, are taken away from home, and you may have justified concern about your child's nutrition. When he or she was eating at home, you could be sure your child was adequately fed; now, it is out of your control. You may find that even though your youngster is eating reasonable, balanced meals at home, he or she is still gaining weight. This means outside eating.

When your teenager says that he or she has nothing to wear, or "Why don't you ever buy me anything?" the real meaning may be "I can't fit into anything." The normal teenager usually is content to wear a pair of jeans and a T-shirt. You have no doubt heard parents of teenagers ask their children why they never wear something else. On the other hand, the

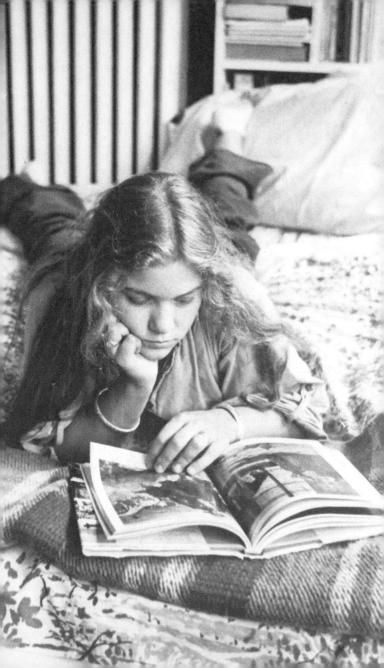

overweight teenager is likely to be constantly looking for something different to wear.

The teenage years are sensitive ones, years in which more attention is paid to looks than to character. It can be a cruel time, because teenagers are apt to judge each other by their clothes, makeup, hair, skin, weight, etc. Far too much emphasis is placed on slimness. Children learn from other children, who learn from their parents.

Teenage values are not mature. Many kids feel that, because they do not have the right "look," they are not as good as their friends. Peer pressure in this age group is very intense. The poor self-image of the overweight teenager only exacerbates his or her food problem; he or she may eat to overcome feelings of worthlessness, not being mature enough to understand that a person's worth is not determined by appearances.

Think back to your teenage years for a minute. I know for myself how important it was to be a member of a group. It probably was for you, too. An overweight teenager may not feel comfortable in any group except, perhaps, a debating society or the school newspaper staff. Being on a prom committee or auditioning for the cheerleading squad are usually out of the question, as are athletic activities and such ordinary teenage pleasures as bike rides or tennis matches. There are exceptions: those teenagers who participate in all that I have mentioned despite their obesity. I am talking about the majority who are crippled by it.

Overweight adolescents may use their obesity to avoid assuming their proper sexual identity. An obese adolescent is less likely to engage in social activities such as school dances, dating, or establishing any normal relations with members of the opposite sex.

A typical scene is that of the overweight adolescent walking around the house with a long face on Saturday night, when everyone else is out on dates or at other social events, saying, "Nobody asked me to go." It may seem that your child is being sullen, or that he or she is antisocial. In reality, the overweight adolescent may be thinking: "I am too fat, and that's why nobody really likes me. I don't want to go out with the other kids; I might be laughed at."

If your teenager is hurting and not going out, you might try to uncover his feelings by asking: "Do you feel uncomfortable about going out with your friends?" Note that I did not suggest that you ask: "Do you feel uncomfortable about your weight?"

It is vital that you keep the lines of communication open between you and your teenager. You must convince him or her that those fatty deposits are merely below the skin and can vanish with proper diet, and that they have nothing to do with character, integrity, or personal worth. A person is to be judged for what he or she is, and not for how he or she happens to look, either in weight, hairstyle, dress, or any other trappings.

Weight reduction in adolescents involves far more than just the loss of weight. Coincidental to the weight loss may be changes in personality, in social life, and in the general outlook of the person. We are thus dealing not only with the body, but also with the mind. Some adolescents may not be prepared for these changes.

Constructive communication between you and your teenager will help to make your child's passage from obesity to slimness a safe, calm, and sound one. Instead of instilling guilt in your child, you can, with effort and love, instill confidence.

It is especially important that you encourage your teenager to make proper food choices. In this way, you can help prepare, him or her to accept responsibility for good nutrition as an adult.

It is not true, as is commonly believed, that teenagers do not like structure. It may seem that way because they are so rebellious. But teenagers are not adults, and they are very much in need of guidance in every area of their lives.

Here are some helpful hints for those teenagers who eat at fast-food establishments:

1. A regular hamburger (minus the top of the bun) and a small bag of French fries have approximately 400 calories. Fast-food is not necessarily *bad* food. We must keep in mind that fast-food establishments cater especially to teenagers. Having an occasional meal at one of these places is important to your child's social

life. Teenagers meet at these places, not only to eat, but also to talk and laugh. For these reasons, your teenager should certainly be allowed to eat there with the proviso that he or she promise not to overindulge.

2. A slice of pizza minus the heavy end crust has about 350 calories and is quite nutritious. Again, there is no reason why this food cannot be incorporated into a teenager's daily diet.

3. Ice-cream parlors are the favorite of all teenage spots, and by far the easiest to work with calorically: usually one scoop of any flavor will not run more than 175 calories. A cone adds an additional 25 to 30 calories, paying high dividends in enjoyment for the relatively small caloric intake.

CHAPTER 4
The Food Link
between Parent and Child

In raising children, parents take on a vast number of responsibilities. The parent hopes to raise a happy, productive human being, who will be emotionally and physically healthy.

Feeding is instinctive on the part of mother or father. A wailing baby elicits immediate attention. If there are no wet diapers or open safety pins, if the room is not too hot or too cold, the parent is most likely to think: "Oh, dear! My baby must be hungry!" Some pediatricians believe that a baby should not be put on a regular feeding schedule; while others advise feeding strictly by the clock.

I, myself, do not remember whether I cried as a baby because I was hungry, because I wanted to be held, or because I wanted my diaper changed. Perhaps I was only crying for the sake of crying. I do not know. The only ways to communicate with my parents were smiles, coos, or red-faced cries. I do not think anyone can scientifically prove exactly why a baby cries at any given moment. I do know from my experience with my own child that a bottle or breast, given tenderly at the right moment, can do wonders to soothe and comfort a distressed infant.

If I were able to become a baby for a few days, and were given my choice of all the activities available to me, such as being rocked, bathed, dressed, powdered, etc., I think I would choose being fed. Why? Being fed carries many warm, comforting overtones in my memory. Father or Mother would hold me close. I would obtain the oral gratification we all need. They would pat me on the back to burp me, and I would feel loved. They would be tender with me, and hold my head carefully as they put me down after my feeding.

Although it is traditional that the mother is the primary giver of food, we must realize that a father's attention to the basic physical needs of his infant is equally important.

Most of us have had this intimate exchange with our parents when we were infants. Thinking of this can give us some clues as to the association between emotion and food formed very early in life.

Since the infant cannot verbalize needs directly, it chooses a medium of communication which provokes the most immediate response. If that response from the parents has been the giving of food, an intelligent baby might learn that it has only to scream to have its parents run to its side with comfort. For many of us, as for me, this comfort came in the form of something to eat, and this food-love association remains to this day. Food means warmth, love, closeness; this is true for most of us.

Becoming aware of your own thoughts and emotions about eating will help you to understand your child's.

By the time the child learns to verbalize needs, the parents may well have learned to pacify the child with a feeding. This pattern of responding on the part of the parent may continue as the child grows older. How many times have you seen a toddler crying, only to have the mother or father give the child a cookie to quiet him or her? The cookie may have been eaten or dropped, intentionally or unintentionally, but, in any case, there is a moment's peace. The child has been pacified—with *food*.

As the child grows up, the parent may use food as a means of disciplining the youngster. For example, the child's reward for learning to use the toilet may be a treat of some sort, usually starch or sugar. By such a response, a parent may build an association in the child's mind between good behavior and food. Mother may say, "You have been such a good girl. Here's a lollipop." This can reinforce the child's notion that emotion is expressed by giving or eating food.

The use of food as a reward creates confusion in a child's mind. The parent, in rewarding successful toilet training with a food treat, may think that the child is delighting in learning self-control. Actually, the child may have no interest in self-control and may only be looking forward to the next lollipop. Food has become something more than what it is: it has become a reward, a punishment, or a pacifier. It has, in short, become a *tool*.

Let us examine more closely the relationship between food, parent, and child. Food becomes an instrument used by the parent for a variety of purposes.

PARENT TO CHILD:

1. "Since you have misbehaved, you will have to go to bed without supper." Here the parent is depriving the child of food as a means of *punishment*.

In later years, the child's association of food with punishment may lead to eating everything quickly, lest it be taken away. Excessive amounts of food may be consumed to forget the memory of hunger when food was denied. Some adults still carry this pain and overeat to compensate for their childhood pangs. Keep in mind that food is powerful. Without food, death is inevitable. Try to find alternative but equally effective punishments, such as: curtailing television privileges or withholding allowances.

2. "If you behave yourself and do not cry when the doctor gives you an injec-

33

tion, I promise to buy you your very favorite ice cream." Here the parent is using food as a *bribe*.

In later years, this connection may lead the child to overeat before a fearful or anxiety-producing situation: for example, a box of cookies eaten before a final exam, or a pint of ice cream consumed before visiting the dentist. The association of unpleasant experiences being ameliorated with food remains deeply embedded in the child's mind through life. Start now by talking honestly about the upcoming event. Yes, it is true that an injection hurts. Explain that the pain is only momentary. Imagine how frightened you would feel at having a knife put into your arm. That is how a child may perceive a needle. Expressing understanding and giving reassurance will serve equally as well as offering food.

3. "I am so delighted with your report card that I will let you have two desserts tonight." In this example the parent is using food as a means of *reward*.

In later years, this association of food with reward may very well backfire. One of the reasons that so many people have a chronic problem in trying to diet is that they tend to reward themselves for staying on their diets by giving themselves the very thing they have denied themselves: food. This is, of course, self-defeating.

The overweight child may be conditioned to expect a reward of food after completing a task successfully. I once had a little patient, a 6-year-old boy, who said that he always went to get a cookie after he hung up his clothes. The parent, in this case, did not give the reward: the child did it himself. Imagine what problems this boy will have in later years, accustomed as he is to this sort of merit system. Even as an adult, it is possible that for every small accomplishment he will reward himself with food. With every treat will come added weight. He is on the way to building a great need to literally and figuratively "feed" his self-esteem.

There are many ways for a parent to reward a child. A reward in the form of hugging or verbal acknowledgement of a job well done can be more meaningful than candy. A bonus at allowance time is an appreciated reward. I have found that giving a child an additional responsibility, one which is pleasurable, is most effective. Your choice of reward should feed your child in another way: he or she should feel more adult and gain a better self-image. Rewarding with food will not accomplish this, but giving love, verbal approval, or a new responsibility will.

> 4. "I am so sorry that your team lost the ball game. Go into the kitchen and cut yourself a nice piece of chocolate cake and have a glass of milk. It'll make you feel better." Here the parent is using food as a means of *consolation*.

Eating as a means of gaining consolation

35

may result in the common practice of consuming food to overcome negative feelings. To prevent this I recommend that consolation be given realistically. A child can be terribly disappointed that his or her team lost the game. It is up to the parent not to soothe with a piece of cake, but to try to change the child's thinking about the loss. Instead of handing out sweets, how much better it would be to empathize with the child and to implant hope that next time the team may win. This kind of communication, direct and to the point, lays a good foundation for later years.

> 5. "Since you're home sick today and you're really not feeling well, I have prepared some yummy chocolate pudding and bought your favorite marshmallow cookies." Here, the parent is using food as a means of *comfort*.

In later years, this pattern of taking comfort in food will be one of the major obstacles to be overcome by the now-adult heavyweight. If a child grows up being given marshmallow cookies every time he or she has a cold, it can be expected that as an adult he or she will follow the same pattern. This practice of giving comfort by giving food is deeply ingrained in our culture, but there are many satisfactory substitutes. A parent can offer comfort by reading to a sick child, playing games with him or her, or simply by spending time with the child. Meaningful social interaction between parent and child is an art that, because of the increasing depersonalization of our society, has deteriorated in many families. Rather than give of themselves, too many parents offer a sweet treat. It is no wonder that childhood obesity and other emotionally caused disorders are on the increase.

> 6. "I know what it's like to lose a friend and how terrible you must feel. I'll make you a homemade hot fudge sundae. It'll help the tears go away." Here the parent is using food as an *emotional pain reliever*.

In later years, the association between food and relief from emotional pain is very hard to erase in the adult mind. Food does not relieve pain; it can only mask it. Attempting to soothe pain with ice cream will only add weight. It will not deal with the problem at hand. Helping the child face pain, acknowledge it, and overcome it is the task of the parent. In this way the child can grow into an adult able to constructively handle pain, rather than masking it compulsively with food. All of us must learn that feeling pain is a part of life and must be dealt with realistically.

There are many ways of disciplining, motivating, soothing, comforting, showing disapproval, and praising. *Food must never be used as a tool under any circumstances*. Food should be presented to the child as a source of nutrition which leads to a sound body and mind. Granted there are times, such as birthday parties or other special occasions, when starches and sweets are traditionally appropriate in limited amounts. An individual does not become fat from celebrating such occasions. It is those in between, everyday indulgences we are concerned with.

I specifically used carbohydrates in the above examples to dramatize the fact that sweets and starches are central to the problem a parent faces with an overweight child. Do you remember your parents telling you that you had to finish your vegetables before you could eat your dessert? That is why desserts become so significant. You may have been conditioned to think that sweets were very special foods, and perhaps that eating vegetables and salads was only a means of getting to the "best" part of the meal, the dessert.

It is very difficult to help an obese child whose brothers or sisters do not have a weight problem. The siblings have free access to the kitchen. The obese child also wants to have that freedom, but cannot handle it without gaining weight. I am against depriving other members of the family of the foods that create problems for the obese child, as I am totally opposed to just telling the troubled child, "You have a weight problem and you are not allowed in the kitchen." There is a way to solve this dilemma. I have suggested this solution often in my counseling sessions and have found it highly successful.

The child is given a very special, large food container with his or her name on it, which is kept in the refrigerator. The parents keep this box filled with low-calorie vegetables, a few cookies, a few slices of cheese, and a very few thin pretzel sticks. During the initial counseling session, the child is told about this box which is to be filled only once a day. It is the child's decision whether to eat all the contents at once or to take small portions throughout the day until it is empty.

Most of the children I work with choose to go to their box throughout the day. That way they feel like "one of the gang" because now they can go into the kitchen and find something to eat for themselves. These children are losing weight and are physically very healthy. But just as important, they are emotionally happy because they do not feel deprived of "refrigerator rights" when they see their siblings marching in and out of the kitchen.

There are some parents who believe in three square meals a day, period. They enforce this rigidity on their children while they allow themselves a mid-morning coffee break, a before-dinner cocktail, and a snack before bed. The child receives a mixed message: "Do as I say, not as I do" — truly bewildering for the child. Children are no less human than adults, and they have a great need for consistency.

By imposing such a rigid schedule for meals, the parents may be inviting rebellion in later years. As the child grows older, he or she could easily act out against this too-strict parental supervision by proclaiming, "Now I can eat whenever I feel like it." This attitude engenders obesity.

On the other hand, no controls at all are just as bad. We must try to find a middle ground, a golden mean, a comfortable and above all *workable* method for dealing with the problem. I cannot emphasize enough the necessity of communicating with your child. Each child is different, and the guidelines for structuring eating habits which I set forth in this book are only general suggestions.

Through the proper use of food and by helping the child form healthy attitudes towards nutrition, a parent can do much to prevent or overcome obesity in a child. In dealing with a child's problem of being overweight, it is essential that you work with your child in tandem with your physician, and that you listen to the youngster. If he or she is forced into a weight-reduction plan, it will not work. You know your child best, and it is only through constant effort and communication that you will come to what is, for both of you, a suitable and effective reducing plan.

Let me give a small example. Many of us tend to equate dieting with no frills and no snacks, almost utter starvation. I disagree with this unyielding attitude. There is no harm in snacking: some children even need between-meal snacks, since they may metabolize faster than others. For the obese child, the danger is not in snacking, but rather in the kinds of food taken as snacks. It is up to the parent to provide nutritious, attractive snack foods for the child. Snacks can be enjoyable foods which will not only contribute to weight loss, but will also be a part of a healthy diet and will help establish sound eating patterns for the future. Some suggestions for such snacks will be found in Chapter Eight.

If an overweight child were to write to us concerning what was needed in order to have the pleasant experience of losing weight, we might receive such letters as these:

Dear Mom and Dad,

Thank you for realizing that I need your help in trying to lose weight. I have been sad for a long time, but I know now that, with a lot of work and with your support, I can feel very happy someday.

I would like to tell you how you can help me with my eating problem.

There are many things which you tell me I must do. Some of these I do not like, but I know that you know best. I may not always like to go to sleep at 9 o'clock, but I know that 9:00 is my bedtime. I know also that I am allowed to watch television for a half hour each school-night and that I may watch it for an hour on weekend nights. Even though I do not like these rules (I would like to watch more TV), I know that I must follow them.

You have told me that I must wear my good clothes to school and my play clothes when

I am in the park or in the yard. I know I must change clothes, even though I don't like to.

I also know that I must write thank-you notes when I get presents from people. I don't like to do this, but, again, I know I must.

These rules you have set up for me help me know what to do. If I did not have your rules to follow, and the rules of the school, I would get very confused. I am learning how people do things, and I need a lot of advice and structure in my life.

There is one thing I do not understand. I do not know when and how I should eat. I wish I had some rules and regulations about the kitchen. I don't know when it is snack time, and I don't know when it's time to eat a real meal. As you know, Mom and Dad, my appetite is not like yours. I don't understand it, either. It's crazy. I don't really know when I'm hungry or when I'm full. I guess, if nobody stopped me, I would just eat all day.

Could we get together and make a schedule for me, so I would have more of an idea about what I should eat and when I should eat it? I think I'd be more comfortable if we sat down and wrote it out and put it on the fridge. We could set times for breakfast, snacks, and dinner on schooldays. On weekends, breakfast would be later, so I could sleep late. Also, you know that desserts are a big problem for me. Wouldn't it be a good idea to have a place on the schedule beside each dinner hour where I could put down when I wanted to have my dessert? Sometimes I like it right after dinner, but waiting until an hour or so later gives me a little treat to look forward to.

I have trouble at night. Maybe it would be good if I promised not to go into the kitchen after I've had dessert. Or, maybe, if I was really hungry, I could ask you what I could have—maybe some carrots. I would be sure not to take anything without asking you first.

What I'm trying to say is that I want you to give me a framework. I am much more comfortable when I know what to do. Once I know I have to do something, it helps me discipline myself. I would rather be told; I can't make up my own schedules yet, at least not with food. It's strange—I can do other things pretty well, but food I just can't handle.

Please, Mom and Dad, let's get together and talk about this. I would like to know what everybody in the family thinks would be good for me—for all of us. I like our family conferences. They make me feel a part of what is going on. A lot of times I feel sort of funny because I am so fat. When we get together and really talk, it assures me that you care about me and will stand by me.

I know that my eating upsets you. It upsets me, too. I don't mean to make you upset or angry. It's just that I don't seem to know my own stomach or appetite very well. Please help. Thanks.

I love you.

Kathleen

43

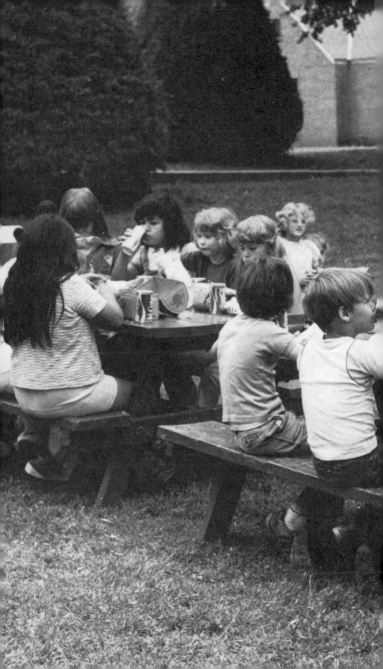

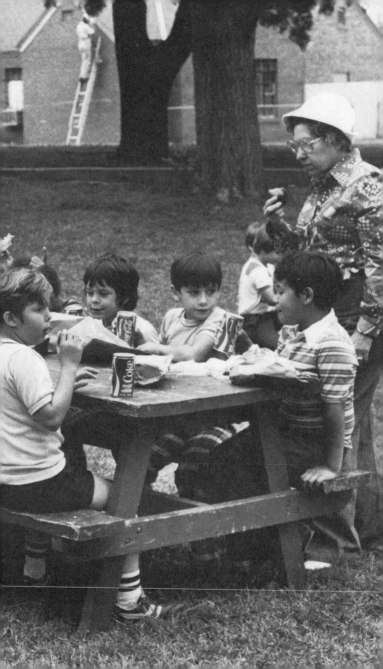

A child might express fear of a difficult situation with these words:

Dear Mom and Dad,

I am scared and I don't know what to do. I'm very excited about going to Bob's birthday party next week. He's my best friend, and a lot of my other friends will be there. What I'm scared of is that I know his Mom is going to bake a big, gooey chocolate cake and special brownies. I love those things. I know, for sure, that there will be ice cream and all kinds of candies and other sweets. You told me that I could have a little ice cream and maybe one cookie. But I know what's going to happen. It does every time, even though I try my best not to let it. I won't be able to control myself, and I'll eat too much of all the wrong things. I can't help it; do you understand that? I don't mean to be bad when I do that, but you scold me when I come home, and I feel terrible.

This makes me feel like not going at all. It'll just be a lot of trouble for all of us because of the food.

I went up to my room and thought about what I could do about this problem. I have an idea. Will you help me with it? I looked at that calorie book you gave me, and I think I have a picture of what 1,000 calories looks like. Suppose we did this: every time I go to a birthday party where there will be all kinds of things I shouldn't eat, we first go to the grocery store and buy lots of popcorn, pretzels, and raisins. If I took these with me, I could have a cup of popcorn for 25 calories, 50 Mister Salty Veri-Thin Pretzel Sticks for 50 calories, and ten raisins for 25 calories. This would be a treat for me, and I could make up little bags the same as mine to take with me to give to all the other kids. That way, I wouldn't feel out of place, and I would be contributing something to the party, too. Would you go to the store with me and buy some of those plastic bags with the twists to close them? I think this would help me out, so I could have a good time at the party with all the other kids, see my best friend, and not get in trouble with the food. Then you wouldn't scold me. If you'll help me, I promise to try my best.

Love,
Craig

Another child might express concern over a different eating problem in the following way:

Dear Mom and Dad,

You know what drives me crazy? It's when I watch TV on Saturday mornings. Those commercials all want you to buy food. They are all trying to sell things like cookies and candies and those cereals with all that sugar on them and chocolate drinks and things that I know I'm not supposed to eat. When I see all these things

47

WHEN YOUR CHILD IS OVERWEIGHT

on the TV, it makes me want to run into the kitchen and get something sweet.

I know how important it is for me to lose weight. You know that I want this more than anything in the world. But sometimes, I don't seem to be able to stop myself from eating. When I eat one cookie, I can't stop. Things like apples and vegetables are much easier for me to handle. I thought it might be a good idea if I ate an apple before I watch TV. That way, I wouldn't be so hungry.

Please tell me what you think of my idea.

Love,
Barry

We can identify other problems in the following hypothetical letter:

Dear Mom and Dad,

I am sorry if I hurt your feelings yesterday morning, but I was feeling bad. Do you remember when I came down to the kitchen, all happy, and said that I had lost two pounds, and then you said: "Let me check on that"? Right then and there, I felt that you didn't trust me. That was bad enough, but when you insisted on seeing the scale in the bathroom with me, I really got mad.

It reminded me of that time when there was a sandwich missing, and, instead of asking Barbara or David if they'd eaten it, you immediately pointed at me and said: "It must have been you." That made me feel terrible, especially since Dad was the one who ate it.

If you could trust me a little more from now on about my weight problem and eating, it would make me feel really good. It's funny, but sometimes when I feel bad, it makes me feel better if I eat something. It's the same when I feel good. When I lost those two pounds and felt so good about it, I kind of wanted to go downstairs and start eating, but I didn't. I was too happy about my weight loss. It seems whenever I feel really bad or really happy, I want to eat. I don't know why.

Love,
Kermit

An overweight child who felt left out of the family might express herself this way:

Dear Mom and Dad,

There's something that really bothers me, and I'd like you to know about it. When Dad goes to the bakery after church on Sunday, and brings home all those good things for the family, he never brings anything for me. He always says that I have to have special food. That makes me feel different.

I asked my teacher in school if there was anything in the bakery I could have that would be lower in calories than the prune Danish and brownies that Dad brings home. She suggested that I might have a bagel. I love bagels. She also said I could have a corn or a blueberry muffin, or maybe a plain doughnut without any sugar on top.

Dad, when you go to the bakery next Sunday, could you get me something, too? It would make me feel a lot better.

Thanks for understanding.

Love,
Ellen

Overweight children undergo considerable trauma in other areas of their lives—not only in dealing with food. A child troubled by her figure might say the following:

Dear Mom and Dad,

I hate to go into the chubby department. It's awful for me to go shopping. It makes me feel very sad. The other day, I was looking through a pattern book at the dime store. I saw some really neat things I know would look super on me until I lose some weight. My girlfriend's mother said it would be less expensive to buy the material and make some new clothes than it would be to buy things at the department store. Boy, I'd feel a lot better if I never had to go into that chubby department again. Clothes are pretty important to me now. I want to look my best. I found out that I could help make my own clothes by putting on the buttons and sewing the hems. Could we do that, please? It would be fun!

Love,
Elizabeth

Children are wonderfully creative when they are allowed the freedom to be so. Allow your child to be involved in all the facets of a weight-loss program. You will find that it will be easier for both of you if you keep the lines of communication open.

CHAPTER 5
Parental Feelings and Relationships

I have devoted most of my attention to your child in the previous chapters of this book. It is now time for you to receive equal attention.

You may have found that your child's weight problem has created tension in your marital relationship. There is often a difference of opinion between parents as to how to treat the troubled youngster. One parent may feel that permissiveness is in order, while the other insists on strictness. It is vital that you consult one another and agree on a mutually acceptable plan of action before embarking on a weight-loss program. In unity there is strength, and through that strength comes the mutual support which is so important in times of stress.

A couple may be reluctant to share their fears about their child's weight problem, thinking that they will be considered intolerant.

Holding back feelings, especially those as strong as the feelings of parent toward child, inevitably results in an explosion which accomplishes nothing.

To aid you, I have made up a list of questions for you to answer. Try to be honest with yourself: it is the only way to help yourself and your child. It might be helpful to record your responses.

1. Have you ever wondered why you could not be like the rest of your friends and have your children draw positive rather than negative reactions?

2. Do you sometimes feel embarrassed when others stare at your child?

3. Do you make excuses for your youngster being overweight by stating that there is a glandular problem?

4. Have you denied your own weight problem, if you have one?

5. Do you look for ways to rationalize your child's weight problem, such as: "My spouse comes from a large-boned family"?

6. Do you sometimes wish the problem would just vanish by itself because you are so sick and tired of it?

7. Do you sometimes despair, feeling that your child will always be overweight, no matter what you may do about it?

If you have answered "yes" to any of the above questions, you will be happy to know that you are a perfectly normal parent! You may not feel comfortable with your affirmative answers, but you should be reassured in knowing that these feelings are not at all uncommon. The more honest you can be with yourself and with your spouse, the better you will be able to cope.

You must be prepared for fluctuations in your child's progress. There will be days and even weeks when everything goes perfectly; there will be others when everything seems to fall apart. In these difficult times, you may feel that your child is being unfair towards you in light of the tremendous amount of effort and energy you are devoting to his or her welfare. It may seem that the child is trying to sabotage your every move. You may feel disappointed and hurt. Rather than immediately expressing your anger, take a few moments to reflect.

Not only should you turn to your spouse in such troubled times, but also be sure to share honestly with your child. Express how you are feeling; be free to vent your frustrations at not understanding why the diet suddenly failed. Accept and express your feelings, but don't blame your child. Ask your child why there was a failure. Try to understand and accept the fact that your child is probably as frustrated as you are.

It is not uncommon for parents of normal weight to have two children, one who is normal and one who is obese. This situation makes it difficult for you to understand your child's problem, since you yourself cannot feel what it is like to be overweight. We are best able to understand another's feelings if we can empathize, and true empathy can come only from having had similar experiences. You therefore should seek help in learning about the dynamics of excessive eating.

Some hospitals around the country have programs for the overweight that are similar to the weekly family conferences in the coronary care unit. It has been felt for some time that the spouse of the heart-attack victim needs to identify with the fears and problems which will arise upon the discharge of his or her partner. Similarly, the spouses of alcoholics, who undergo the trauma of living with a sick person, can obtain help in dealing with their problems by going to Al-Anon, while the afflicted party attends Alcoholics Anonymous. Weight control clinics or counselors often provide such a service for those afflicted with obesity.

Books are a good source for gaining some understanding of compulsive eating. Publications such as *The Story of Weight Watchers**, by Jean Nidetch; *How to Be A Thin Person*, by Raysa Rose Bonow; and one of my earlier works, *The Freedom Diet—Games Dieters Play*, are all informative and provide you with valuable insights into what it is like to have a weight problem. Any biographical work which gives you a glimpse into the world of the troubled eater will be of great value to you.

You may not be able to empathize with the exact feelings of the compulsive eater, but you can identify with not being able to gain

*For publication information on this and other works listed, see page 95.

control of a problem situation. The more you are able to get in touch with your feelings, the more you will be able to cope with your child's.

I myself was an overweight teenager. I had initially thought that I would include here some of my own painful experiences in being obese. I reconsidered. This book is primarily about the overweight *child*, not the overweight adolescent.

There is nothing positive about being overweight. Yes, I feel for the parent, but it is the child who suffers the most from obesity, and I do not believe that anyone who has not been through this childhood affliction has any idea of what it feels like. There is real pain involved. I decided the best way to communicate this pain would be to include firsthand accounts of individuals who were overweight as children.

The first story was written by a young man now working in New York. He grew up overweight, and is now battling the problem as an adult. I think he will succeed. I will say no more, for his words speak for themselves.

"At the age of three, my family moved to Puerto Rico. We spent the next three-and-one-half years there. We moved back to New York City when I was seven.

"Moving three thousand miles is a big shift in anyone's life. I had already spent two years of my life with the kids in my school and I was now about to be dropped into a room with thirty strangers who had spent the same portion of their lives together. The same thing happened when my parents uprooted me from my home and friends in junior high school and college.

"I don't think it's coincidence that my weight problem mushroomed at the age of seven. I found solace in food and television. I spent more time absent from school than any person I have ever known: forty days in a year was not unusual. Recalling it now, I guess this was all with my mother's approval. I would wake up and say, 'I don't feel good.' My father would say in a hushed tone to my mother (but always loud enough to be overheard): 'He's faking.' And Mommy would reply, 'Just let him stay home today.' I almost always won out—the loss to my early life was monumental.

"The day home from school always contained plenty of TV and plenty of food. I was wise enough to know that faking an upset stomach was to be kept to a minimum. Sometimes I sacrificed the day's food intake so when my father got home, my mother would tell him: 'He really must be sick; he didn't eat all day.' This was usually good for the next two days, during which I would, of course, eat frantically.

"Food and television are inextricably linked in my mind; today the television always seems to be on when I'm having a binge. My mother always connected the two; if a special program was on, that meant something 'really nice to eat.' Going to the store was always dependent upon what TV show was on. I grew up thinking of TV and food as my only two friends.

"Obviously, if your best friends are television and the refrigerator, it cuts down on your social life. It is still a very real pain to be the only person not to get a Valentine, or to be one of the few people not invited to a party given by one of your classmates. The few times I invited someone over, my mother immediately overwhelmed them with potato chips and cookies and soda and the like. It's only now that I've come to realize that not everybody constructs their life as rigidly around food as I had mine: our dinner conversation was always about what was for dinner tomorrow!

"There was only one conclusion to draw from my schoolmates' dismay at my life: rather than accept the fact that it was my home life that was weird, I concluded that my classmates were somehow inferior to me. Since I never fully accepted this notion, my mind became more twisted and confused, and I retreated further into the only comfort I knew: pigging out in front of the television set. The worse the pain, the more I aggravated it: *Catch 22*, even if I didn't understand it back then.

"All I can add about my life as a fat kid is a simple declarative sentence: IT WAS HORRIBLE!"

The following story was written by a young woman who also had the problem of childhood obesity. I again shall say no more, except to thank both these fine people for their honesty and courage in revealing such very personal information.

"Until I reached the sixth grade, being a fat kid wasn't bad. It didn't seem to affect the way I felt about myself nor my relationships with other people. I was lucky, because I was popular in school. I was good in schoolwork and good in kickball, and I was a leader in almost everything. Besides, there were always two or three girls who were a lot fatter than I was. I wasn't uncomfortable with my body, I wasn't left out of things, and I wasn't afraid to take part in activities because of embarrassment. I didn't think of my fat as a problem.

"Sixth grade brought the change. My school gave us a mid-morning snack of juice, milk, or a sandwich, depending on what our parents ordered. My mother ordered only juice for me, because sandwiches were 'fattening.' This shows that by this time my parents saw my weight as a problem and were trying to do something about it. I remember I used to hang around the food tray and eat the sandwiches my thin friends didn't want. I probably ate two or three halves every day. I remember feeling a tremendous *need* to have the sandwiches, which may have been partly physical but which was mainly emotional.

"Several emotions began to be connected with food. There was a strong feeling of guilt, because I knew I wasn't supposed to have the sandwiches. There was a feeling of embarrassment, of being afraid that people would notice how much I was eating. (I was careful to ask a different set of friends each day.) Finally, there

59

was a feeling of excitement, almost of glee! I was tricking *them*! I was managing to eat despite all *their* efforts!

"All these feelings grew stronger as I grew up. Food summoned up these feelings, and these feelings led me to food. Getting food and eating it without being caught became one of the major activities of my life. As a kid, being fat was simply a physical problem. In sixth grade, it became an emotional one, and that was the crucial point. It was then that I wished things could be different.

"I don't recall any scenes at the dinner table when I was younger. Mainly, I remember having a feeling of fury when I was told not to eat something, a surge of anger that colored all other areas of my life with my family. It increased my desire to defy my parents, to eat what was forbidden, even though I was really only hurting myself. We never had things like cake or bread in the house: we hardly ever had desserts. My father always cooked with few fats, and served mainly vegetables and meat. I had little opportunity to overeat at home, and therefore I started to go out and buy things. I became a very secretive kid. I had to eat what I brought home in the bathroom or in my closet. I had to hide the containers from my parents, even going so far as to throw the empty containers away on my way to school. I developed secret personal habits, all relating to food, and these started to affect the way I acted with other people in things completely unrelated to food. My guilt about eating grew until I started to think of myself as a totally guilty person.

"I started to block off areas of my life which couldn't be shared with other people, because if they ever found out about my secret eating, they would hate me. I kept quiet about my problems with food, and I started to keep quiet about everything else.

"My mother struggled with her weight all her life, and my brother and sister have weight problems, although theirs didn't develop until they were older. Since we normally didn't have fattening things in the house, we grew up with the attitude that whenever we had a party or went out to dinner, we might as well stuff ourselves, because we weren't going to see those foods for a long time. My family centered its rituals around food: Thanksgiving, Christmas Eve dinner, and Christmas lunch. Vacations in Vermont became associated with uncontrolled binges, because in Vermont my mother bought all the foods we never had at home. License to eat ice cream and cake brought with it license to eat huge amounts of everything else. There was and is no control of portions in our house. If a cake is in the icebox, it is gone in a few minutes; each person trying to take as big a piece as possible, because if he doesn't take it the first time, he'll never get any more. A feeling of excitement is still attached to certain foods, a feeling of delightful sinfulness which overcomes any negative feelings about gaining weight. I learned to have this feeling, and I wish I had

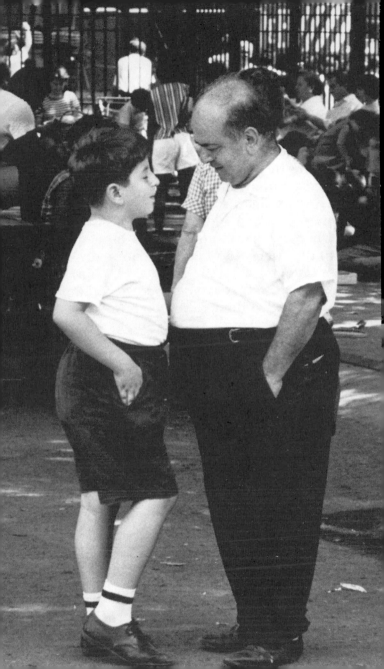

learned instead to treat every kind of food equally, with detachment rather than hysteria.

"As I got older, life became a series of horrible events which I had to live through, horrible only because I was fat. I started to be left out of parties and dances. Dancing school was hell, because no boy wanted to dance with me. The greatest day of my life was March 8, 1968, which was the last time I had to go to dancing school. Finding clothes was hell, and nothing looked good on me. Time after time, I remember crying in the dressing room because I finally had to face my fat.

"Two events stand out in my mind. In seventh grade, Mom took me shopping for a spring coat, and it was hard to find anything. A saleslady said, to comfort me: 'It's just baby fat. You'll grow out of it,' and my mother answered sharply: 'It's not baby fat—she could lose it if she'd only try.' I knew she was really speaking to me, not to the saleslady. I remember being terribly ashamed that she had said something like that in front of a complete stranger. I was furious at her for not caring about my feelings.

"Another time, Mom bought me an orange knit shirt, a color I detested, and when I tried it on at home, I said to her that the color made my skin look yellow. She said to me: 'Honestly, no one's going to even notice your skin, the way you look.' The feelings of despair and anger are as strong in me now as I write this, as they were then.

"So, starting in sixth grade I learned

that the only thing that matters in life is how you look. I could be bright in school and a charming conversationalist, but this was worth nothing as long as I was fat. I felt that people would take an interest in me only if I was thin, and I learned to be angry at men for caring only about my body. Today my whole feeling of self-worth depends on how other people see me, so I have to act in ways that will make people like me. My body image has become my whole self-image.

"I wish that somehow something had been done when I was ten to stop this cycle. I don't know what could have been done, just that what *was* done was obviously not right. If I ever have a child with a weight problem, I will try to do two things: I will try as hard as possible to give my child a strong sense of confidence in him- or herself that is not dependent upon physical appearance. I will try to teach that the body is only a part, an important part, but not the whole being. Secondly, I will try to instill in my child a relaxed attitude towards food—to see it as neither an enemy nor a friend. I will try to keep food as free from emotions as I can, so that it does not become a substitute for them. That's what I wish had been done for me."

I hope the foregoing accounts help you realize that an overweight child may have an "appestat" that simply does not function. He or she may be, as these letters exemplify, completely confused about what most of us take for granted: the ability to know when we are hungry, when we are full, when we should eat, and when we should stop.

Essential to your child's progress in weight reduction is your understanding of all his or her difficulties. It is for this reason that you must encourage expression of feelings, not only about food, but about many other things. The more your son or daughter can be made to feel an integral member of the family, a part of the school group, and a valuable human being who is loved and understood, the better the progress will be. Unfortunately, the child with a weight problem is often considered "bad" or "rebellious," not *impaired*. He or she needs the same loving support as another afflicted child. Your special child needs your special care.

CHAPTER 6
From Obesity to Health

Behavior modification is one of the most effective tools used in breaking undesirable habits. It has been used with overweight children whose food intake was excessive. Part of their problem may be simply that they have developed poor eating habits. These may yield to behavior modification. We must attempt to change the behavior of the overweight child with respect to food. In order for this technique to work, we must first set the goals we wish to reach. When a goal is reached, we then reward the changed behavior, thus reinforcing it, and try for the next goal.

You probably have heard of Pavlov's experiment with the dog and bell. Dr. Pavlov would ring a bell every time he set food before his dog. He repeated this procedure time after time, until the dog's association between bell-ringing and food was so strong that salivation occurred upon the sound of the bell, even with no food present.

Human beings, too, are often programmed into certain types of behavior and physiological responses. Many of us, for example, salivate, just as did Dr. Pavlov's dog, when we first sit down to the dinner table. Just the anticipation of eating, since we are accustomed to having food at this time and in this place, is enough to make our salivary glands start working.

Most probably you have had some experiences in trying to break an annoying or even health-threatening habit. Smoking, hair pulling, nail biting, are all difficult to deal with. Overeating is one of the most difficult to overcome.

In dealing with undesirable actions through behavior modification, punishment for bad behavior is much less effective than rewards for good behavior. The compensation for appropriate behavior is called "positive reinforcement."

Let's look at some examples of how this "positive reinforcement" works in a program of weight loss:

Case I

Michael is 11 years old and 20 pounds overweight. The desired weight loss will be divided into 5 pound goals, and every time a loss of 5 pounds is achieved, a reward will be given to reinforce this success.

Initial loss: 140 to 135 pounds—tickets to a sports event or theatrical production.

Second loss: 135 to 130 pounds—trip to amusement park.

Third loss: 130 to 125 pounds—a new volleyball or badminton set, or perhaps a new baseball glove.

Fourth loss: 125 to 120 pounds—a monetary reward, such as a couple of dollars.

You will note that the suggested rewards for Michael's success in losing weight are ones in which the entire family can share, except, perhaps for the slight monetary one, which is a special treat for the child himself. These rewards do not set the child apart from his family setting. They are designed to further his relationships with family members. Child and family can all share in the excitement.

These material rewards are only representations of the best and most effective reward of all. The most precious thing we can give our children in any situation is *love*.

Case II

Pamela is thirteen years old and an only child. She wants to loose 15 pounds. Goals and rewards:

130 to 125 pounds—increase of one dollar per week in allowance.

125 to 120 pounds—new record album.

120 to 115 pounds—new dress.

You will note that these rewards for

Pamela are a bit different than those I suggested for Michael. Pamela is an only child, and there is no need in this case to ensure that the rewards be enjoyed by the entire family. It is important to note that positive behavior is being rewarded, and that negative behavior is not being punished.

There are many ways to set up a behavior modification program in your home and there are various goals you can set. It is very important that you and your child determine together, along with your physician the goals for your child's weight-loss program. It will not succeed if the child sees it as something imposed by the parent. You might determine together a certain length of time in which your child will lose a certain amount of weight. But be careful: if you allot too little time, it might be impossible for your child to attain the goal. He or she may become discouraged. On the other hand, too much time will allow the child to dally at the task, putting it off "until tomorrow," which can be "forever."

I myself prefer the 24-hour contract principle. This means that the child makes a commitment for only 24 hours at a time. This technique is especially valuable when a child is having a particularly difficult time adhering to his or her diet. A commitment could be made to eat only what has been portioned out for that one-day period. If the child fulfills the contract, he or she should be rewarded with smiles, kisses, and an abundance of love. Immediate reinforcement for each successful 24-hour period is essential, in order that your child look forward to another positive reward for his or her behavior on the following day. Be consistent in rewarding the child every single day. You must instill confidence in your child, and this you can do only by being consistent in your behavior and attitude.

Open communication and the sharing of feelings is very important in motivating a child to stay on a weight-loss program.

For example:

PARENT TO CHILD: "How do you feel about the fact that you were able to maintain your diet today?"

CHILD TO PARENT: (almost invariably) "I really feel good about it."

PARENT TO CHILD: "I know you can do it again."

CHILD TO PARENT: "I really think I can, now. It makes me feel so good."

In this sort of interchange, the child is beginning to feel good and thus learning to reinforce his or her own actions. Low self-esteem is most often one of the primary motivating factors behind a child's obesity. When the youngster begins to feel good about him- or herself, he or she will be less likely to overeat. The new experience of feeling good about one's own achievement, coupled with a loss of weight that is properly reinforced, can change a child's whole outlook and build the conviction that success is possible in other areas of life as well.

The child's pattern of thinking will change: Instead of acting out of fear of punishment, the child will act because he or she wants positive reinforcement.

Rewards of love, appreciation, parental closeness, and understanding are always preferable to harshness or punishment. By standing behind your child with encouragement, instead of hovering over him or her with threats, you will not only be encouraging the loss of excess weight, but you will also be establishing a new way of relating to your child which will last for the rest of your lives.

The effective use of support systems can be invaluable to you in seeing a child's weight-loss program through to success. Your child's doctor, the school, your church, and various sources of information can all be most helpful to you.

Your doctor is the best authority to guide you and your child through a weight-loss program. It is he or she who should decide what kind of diet your child should follow, and what vitamins, if any, are to be given. Do not attempt to develop a weight-loss program for your child without a doctor's assistance. Ask for such help as a weekly weigh-in or a special visit—this might encourage your child. You should feel free to telephone your doctor should you have any specific questions. Many parents feel that they should not disturb a doctor except in crisis situations. Although your child may not be suffering physically, the obesity is your child's and your family's pain. Your doctor should support you at all times. If you feel a lack of interest from your physician, re-evaluate your relationship. You are paying the bills.

The school nurse can be of tremendous assistance, particularly in giving support to your child. A weekly visit can be set up for a quick weight check, a friendly smile, and lots of encouragement. You might speak to the principal, the school nurse, and the P.T.A. president about setting up a weight-reducing program in the school. I was asked many years ago to set up such a program for the North Country Elementary School in Stony Brook, Long Island, N.Y. One of the teachers there was concerned about the weight problems of her students: It was thus that the Slimming Club was started. Parents were notified through a school mailing. All children wanting to participate were required to have on file their physician's approval. Our weekly meetings were filled with fun, education, and much success in losing weight. We had no failures, but all rallied behind those who were having difficulties. I did not allow competition, as this can be emotionally damaging to the child who is struggling. The children all shared "tips and tricks." Some of these were better than professional suggestions; I still use them in my sessions.

I also held weekly rap sessions for the parents, so that they could voice frustrations and/or have their questions answered. These meetings were just as important as the ones with the children. Through age eight, children need parental supervision and much directive advice; they are not capable of governing themselves. Educating the parent is essential to the child's success in losing weight. There must be a balance between supervision which is too strict and could cause discomfort, and utter permissiveness, which creates chaos. For this balance, most parents need the help of a professional.

If you feel that you and your child are having difficulty in communicating, your minister, priest, or rabbi may have the answer for you. Spiritual guidance, when there is a problem with patience, will always help. I was asked to give a lecture by the wife of a minister who had an obese child. This resulted in a program similar to the one I had started in Stony Brook. On the bulletin board, one of our "think tank" sheets went as follows:

I, your child, ask you to be firm, but not harsh.

I, your child, ask that you be supportive, not critical.

I, your child, ask that you be sympathetic, not distant.

I, your child, ask that you be tolerant, not demanding.

I, your child, ask that you be compassionate, not scolding.

I, your child, ask that you be active, not passive.

I, your child, ask that you be involved, not disinterested.

I, your child, ask that you be concerned, not angry.

73

I, in turn, will give you all my effort in trying to lose weight.

I, in turn, will thank you for years to come for your strength.

I, your child, will bless you forever for sparing me the pain of an adult weight problem.

Without knowledge, you are powerless to teach. Inadequate information could cause real problems. Learn all you can about nutrition and weight loss. *Dictionary of Nutrition,* * by Richard Ashley and Heidi Duggal is a very easy book to read, and, in my opinion, highly informative. The government publication, *Composition of Foods,* Agricultural Handbook No. 8, is an outstanding publication that lists in dictionary format, the calories, protein, fats, carbohydrates, minerals, and vitamins of various foods. Another outstanding book is *Calories and Carbohydrates,* by Barbara Kraus. This book gives the consumer the calorie and carbohydrate counts of foods according to brand names. A more detailed and definitive work is the *Nutrition Almanac,* published by McGraw-Hill. The knowledge you gain from these works will be of invaluable assistance.

A successful weight-loss program involves not only the overweight child and parents, but also brothers and sisters. The family with a little creative imagination can come up with special family projects that will provide

*For publication information on this and other works listed, see page 95.

added motivation for losing weight. An example of such a project is one I developed called "The Love Project." Since so many children of the world are starving, I thought both severely underweight and overweight children would benefit from this project.

The campaign was named: "Feed a Child and Nourish Your Soul." On one day each month, a family would eat only the bare necessities. The money saved would then be donated to a world hunger project. A family could easily contribute several dollars by this practice. In addition, the children could be taught to happily limit the money they spend on candy, and to donate their nickles and dimes to feed a hungry child. Involve your overweight child in feeling needed and wanted, and you will get a positive response. She or he will be motivated to give up some pleasure in food to nourish a needy sister or brother somewhere in the world.

You must realize that your weight-troubled child probably suffers from low self-esteem. Food has become the means for dealing with feelings which seem overwhelming. By giving food to others, your child can learn to use food in a positive way and at the same time come to feel better about him- or herself. Your child's ego will be bolstered, and perhaps he or she will come to know the meaning of real hunger. No child is too young to understand this translation of food into spiritual nourishment. I remember, thirty years ago, giving up some of my toys to a Red Cross project, so that another child would have a merry Christmas. I cannot remember ever feeling better about giving than at that moment.

Let it be known to your entire family that your child is on a weight-reduction program. Elicit support. If Grandma always brings homemade fudge, you might suggest that she bring apples instead. No one will feel deprived, and all will benefit without a caloric disaster. Thinly-coated, chocolate-dipped bananas are easier on Auntie than making pecan pie, and certainly easier on everyone's diet.

Some advice about brothers and sisters. Invariably, the overweight child feels like an outsider, especially if there are siblings who are of normal weight. It seems cruel to the overweight child to be placed on a special diet, while brothers and sisters munch on anything they wish. Jealousy may set in, along with bitter fights. It is up to the parents to bring the children together in an open family meeting. Your child's weight problem should be discussed as openly as though your child were afflicted with something as obvious as a limp. Teasing a fat child is one of the normal child's most vicious weapons. Show that teasing is cruel, and that your normal-weight children would certainly not want to be picked on for whatever they may feel bad about in themselves.

Think of family projects that would involve your overweight child. Togetherness dispels loneliness, and children use food as one of the fillers for loneliness—as do many adults.

CHAPTER 7
Toward a New Self-Identity

The transition from obesity to health may prove to be quite difficult. It would seem natural for a child who has reached a weight-loss goal to be quite happy about it. This is true in the majority of cases. But there are those who experience this change as trauma. Let us look at this minority.

There is a period of adjustment to the new body, and this can cause an identity crisis, especially for the child whose obesity is of long duration. The child who has been overweight for a long time may react to the radical change in his or her body by withdrawing. He or she has had an identity based on being fat: now that this condition no longer exists, the child no longer feels like the same individual. He or she may face an identity crisis, uncertain of the new image.

You, as a parent, can understand this difficulty from your own experience. It is like any other transition. We have all been through major life-changes, such as leaving home, getting married, going into the real world after leaving the shelter of school. Do you remember how you felt when suddenly you were no longer under the protection of your parents, but had to stand on your own as an adult? We all have had times when we did not know where we belonged or exactly who we were. It is this feeling that some obese children experience upon weight loss.

You may even find your child quite depressed and uneasy. Terrifying thoughts such as: "Is part of me dead? Where did I go? I am a stranger to myself. I am scared. . . ." may trouble the youngster. Other children will be elated with thoughts such as "I am glad to be the new me. I love my new body. I feel good." Both positives and negatives may occur.

We are talking here about simple human fear. Years ago in one of my courses, I read a paper which dealt with children's fears. The author had chosen to investigate why children cried in the bathtub. The author concluded that: a) The child's perception of his or her body changed when he or she was immersed in the water. Some children enjoyed the bouyancy; others were frightened by it. b) The child's fright increased when the tub was drained while the child was still in it. The child's imagination was carrying him or her down the drain with the

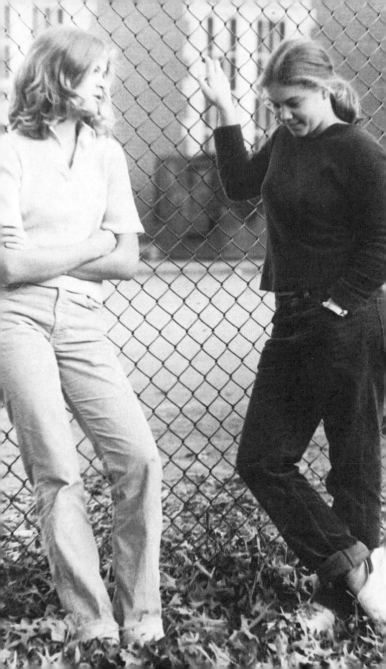

water, and hydrophobia (fear of water) resulted.

Fear of the loss of self is very real. It was then faced at every bath time. A child may react with trauma, as do many adults, to the loss of a tooth or to a haircut. Part of the body is being lost. Anyone who has had even minor surgery, such as a tonsillectomy, knows the sense of loss which occurs when a part of your body is taken from you.

The child who loses a substantial amount of weight can easily experience this as a loss of part of him or herself. He or she may feel weaker, smaller, less powerful. If this is the case, the unconscious need to increase the inner sense of power by increasing body size will lead to a return to excessive eating. The successful weight loss then brings about a weight gain, and the yo-yo syndrome is born, with weight going up or down, but never stabilizing.

You should always reward your child for any job well done. As I have indicated, weight loss can be a delicate process. It is therefore essential that you refrain from any comments which might embarrass the child or have any negative effect. For example, you should *not* say things like: "You are not the same person." "Half of you just disappeared." "You look so different, I didn't even recognize you." These comments might indicate to the youngster that there is something odd about his or her appearance, and that the weight loss is not fully welcomed.

Far better are comments such as: "You look wonderful." "It's so nice to see you smile like that." "Where did you get that pretty dress?" Since there is a possibility that the child may be uncomfortable at first with his or her new body, it might be best to refrain from any remarks on physical matters and keep your conversation in a general vein, making it clear that you accept and love the child for what he or she is, not for what his or her weight happens to be.

Other children are so anxious to stay slim that they may exaggerate their dieting efforts. The fear of returning to an overweight state creates such pressure in the mind that the child may literally begin to starve. This situation may lead to a condition known as "anorexia nervosa." This is a very serious disease in which the child (usually an adolescent at puberty) loses control of body image, reality, and the ability to perceive hunger. Thin is never thin enough. The lower the weight, the further from that ever present demon, the appetite. It was, after all, that larger-than-life appetite which caused those obese days. The goal of life becomes to kill the appetite, ensuring that the obesity will never again occur.

The child loses all sense of how the body looks. (Of all those with anorexia nervosa, 98% are girls.) An arm devoid of muscle, just bone covered with skin, makes us shudder. To the child, however, everything looks normal. Protruding rib cage and hip bones look wonderful. "The less flesh, the safer" becomes the motto.

Parents, relatives, and friends can aggravate this disease in an adolescent. Comments such as: "Of course I loved you when you were overweight, but now that you are thin, I love you more" may be made. A child may think: "The thinner I am, the more loved I will be." Other comments, such as "You look so wonderful, I want to show you off to everyone," can be devastating. The child will come to equate thinness not only with acceptance but adulation. This reinforces the conviction in the youth's mind: the thinner, the better. Recovery from anorexia nervosa is most difficult. Be judicious in your comments about your child's new body. Praise is wonderful when given for the correct reason.

Another disease which has been attributed to weight loss is known as "bulimarexia." This condition is also a nightmare. It is characterized by enormous quantities of food being ingested, followed by periods of voluntary vomiting. As the disease progresses, the vomiting may become uncontrollable. There is such an abnormal fear of gaining weight that the child develops these symptoms as a means of gaining control.

Note: Anorexia nervosa and bulimarexia are said in these instances to be secondary to obesity. In the majority of cases, both diseases occur without any history of obesity.

CHAPTER 8
The Careful Consumer

When I was in school, one of my nutrition education courses dealt with the subject of food merchandising. None of us needs a formal course, however, to realize what an enormous impact the advertising people have on us, often without our awareness. Our food choices are often dictated by the media, and the media do not always have health or nutrition in mind.

I suggest that you make a special trip to your supermarket, just to evaluate it. On this trip, plan not to buy anything. You might even go without money. The purpose of this visit will be to acquaint you with your store in a new way. Try to step out of your usual role of "consumer" and into the role of "observer."

I have found two safe zones in the supermarket. The first is the fresh fruit and vegetable section. These departments carry mostly unprocessed, unadvertised goods, goods with a high turnover. Madison Avenue has not yet invaded the celery stalks or those containers of chicken livers or gizzards which are so nutritious and yet so inexpensive. But high-pressure advertising is, no doubt, one good reason why so many people spend more money than necessary for good protein and vitamin foods. We are told through advertisements which cuts of meat to buy. More often than not, these cuts are overrated and quite expensive. A "well-marbled" slab of meat is supposed to be a real treat for us and something of a status symbol. Here we could use a little education. The protein and vitamin content of those inexpensive chicken gizzards is much higher and the fat content much lower, than that of the expensive piece of advertised meat. Although the meat department is comparatively safe, there are important cautions to be exercised.

Vegetables and fruits are even safer. An apple is an apple, and advertising has not yet been able to influence the purchase of a particular head of cabbage.

The areas of the supermarket in which you must be most careful are those in which you find the processed, packaged items. On this evaluative visit, practice picking up boxes and cans and looking carefully at the labels. Especially when dieting, we must take care to choose wisely and pay strict attention to protein and vitamin intake. Most containers now carry full nutritional information. Since we are restricting our foods, we must be sure to give our bodies what they need. In designing your child's diet, the doctor will outline daily needs. Adequate protein is very important in a diet and it is advisable to keep count of the grams of protein consumed each day. The problem is that many processed foods are low in protein and high in refined starches and sugars.

On this special visit, ask yourself why you choose to pick up particular foods. Is it because you have been brainwashed by the media? Have your children seen an item on television and begged for it? Or is it because something is on sale and you can hardly resist the savings, even though you might not ordinarily buy it? Is it a new product which catches your attention, or might it be that you think your family deserves a special treat?

All these factors contribute to our decisions on what we buy. The pressures can be such that we may tend to ignore those valuable nutritional rundowns on the label. It is your responsibility to give yourself an education in nutrition and to learn to be watchful in the stores, especially when you are in those danger zones where the packages and advertising may beckon you to a product which is nutritionally poor and calorically rich.

For example, when buying cookies for the family, you could make a choice between animal crackers, with about 12 calories each, and Keebler Bavarian Fudge Cookies, with 79 calories each. You might choose Sunshine Arrowroot Cookies at 15 calories apiece, instead of Sunshine Macaroons at 85 each. You could select Keebler Honey Grahams for 17 instead of Keebler Old Fashioned Oatmeal Cookies for 78 calories.

Children usually love crackers. Think of the service you would be doing your child if you were to serve tiny oyster crackers at 3 calories each, instead of Ritz Crackers which have 18 calories each, or if you were to serve Nabisco Wheat Thins at 9 calories, instead of Triscuits with 22 calories?

Breakfast cereals are among the most heavily advertised products on children's TV programming. It can be a real challenge to your parenting skills and to your ability as a careful shopper to purchase the right cereals.

A spoon-sized Nabisco Shredded Wheat Biscuit yields 4 calories. Twenty of these would yield 80 calories. In my opinion, this is one of the best cereals on the market: it has no sugar, is pure whole wheat, and is quite filling. I recommend it highly.

If you were to buy Post Grape-Nuts, you would be offering 400 calories per cup serving. In contrast, the same amount of Kellogg's Special "K" would have only 70 calories. A poor choice might be Cap'n Crunch Pre-Sweetened Corn Oats, by Quaker, with 163 calories per cup, compared to Kellogg's Corn Flakes which have only 79 calories per cupful.

You may find that your investigatory visit to the supermarket will reveal that your approach to shopping and homemaking has some bearing on your child's weight problem. Let's take an example: One cup of plain Dannon yogurt has about 140 calories, whereas most of the flavored yogurts have between 260 and 270 calories. I suggest that you flavor the yogurt yourself. You could add a teaspoon of jam, 16 calories, to plain yogurt and then have only 156 calories. You will not only save approximately 100 calories but you will also be doing the family budget a favor.

Another example: an eight-ounce glass of 1% skim milk will yield approximately 80 calories, while a glass of whole milk will be about 150 calories. A glass of Carnation Instant Breakfast comes to 290 calories; a six-ounce glass of Heinz canned Apple Juice is a slim 75 calories. The same portion of Welch's Grape Juice, however, is a hefty 128 calories. If you choose to have a six-ounce glass of Heinz canned Grapefruit Juice, your child will be taking in 68 calories, but if you choose the same amount of Dole Pineapple Juice, the calories will be 110.

Let's look at some more choices. Canned Hi-C Punch has 130 calories in eight ounces. You could serve your child twelve ounces of canned vegetable juice for only 70 calories.

When it comes to cheese, you will find 50% fewer calories in low-fat American cheese products. You can purchase low-fat cottage cheese, instead of the 4% kind, for a savings of approximately 30 calories per cup.

Children are very fond of soups. They are easy to prepare, and fill empty stomachs. Here again careful shopping can greatly enhance the success of your child's diet. Let's see what is available. All comparisons are for eight-ounce portions.

Campbell's Turkey Noodle Soup is a good choice—only 75 calories. On the other hand, Campbell's Green Pea Soup at 148 calories is not as wise a choice. Campbell's Mushroom Soup from the can has 80 calories and is a better choice than the same soup prepared with milk, which will have 270 calories.

Vegetables should be served plain. By themselves, either fresh, frozen, or canned, they are not a caloric problem. A few, mostly legumes or tubers, are relatively high in calories. It is only when you buy vegetables in convenience packages, where they may be creamed, au gratin, or in sauces, that there is caloric trouble. For example, half a cup of Campbell's Baked Beans in Barbecue Sauce has 171 calories whereas one-half cup of Birdseye 5 Minute Asparagus Cuts is only 21 calories.

Frozen TV dinners may not be as nutritious as some other foods, but they are very much a part of the American scene, and must be taken into account. One advantage of this type of food is that it is portion controlled. If you add a salad, a piece of fruit, and a glass of skim milk, you will have a fairly decent meal. I would not recommend this for every day, but a couple of times a week would certainly not hurt.

Careful shopping can make a big difference. For example: a 10 ¾-ounce Banquet Beans and Franks Dinner runs a high 687 calories, whereas a 10-ounce Banquet Ham Dinner is only 352 calories. The 11-ounce Banquet Beef Dinner is a sound choice at only 295 calories, whereas the 11-ounce Banquet Fried Chicken Dinner is a poor choice at 542 calories. The 12-ounce Morton Turkey Dinner is a hefty 460 calories; the 11 ½-ounce Banquet Turkey Dinner is only 280. You can see how you can substitute one kind of frozen dinner for another and save calories, or even, as with the turkey dinners, have the same thing and still save calories by choosing different brands.

Pizza is another favorite of children. Buitoni markets an instant frozen cheese pizza, 2 ¾ ounces for 139 calories. Chef Boy-Ar-Dee has the same size frozen cheese pizza for 164 calories. Both of these are good purchases, when you compare them with the Roman 3 ¼-ounce Frozen Sausage Pizza, which has 234 calories.

Does your child like mayonnaise on everything? You could save considerable calories (42%) by buying imitation mayonnaise which tastes about the same. Does he or she rebel at salad without dressing? One tablespoon of oil will cost 100 calories. You might try some of the diet dressings on the market; they are quite tasty and can be as low as 8 calories per tablespoon. You might try making your own diet dressings. Experimenting is fun!

Ketchup is another ubiquitous item in

most children's diets. When your child pours it over everything in sight, he or she is taking in 18 calories with each tablespoon. To cut the calories, I suggest you dilute the ketchup with water, so that the flavor is still there, minus some of the weight-producing calories.

Perhaps your child has a sweet tooth. Your best bet in the cake department is always angelfood cake, carrying the lowest calorie count of any on the market.

If you have a child who insists on those individual little packaged cakes, don't despair. Drake's all-butter Junior Pound Cake, 1.1 ounces, is only 104 calories. Compare this to the 2 ¼-ounce Drake's Devil Dog at 307 calories. New on the market are Durkee Petit Cinnamon Danish Whirls, at only 78 calories each. Think of the calorie saving you would achieve by giving one of these to your youngster instead of, say, a strawberry turnover by Pepperidge Farm for 326 calories.

Pretzels are a favorite American snack. Here again, there is a choice: chooose Nabisco Mister Salty Dutch Pretzels, 51 calories each, or Mister Salty Veri-Thin Pretzel Sticks, only one calorie each!

These examples are only to give you an idea of what you can do by shopping carefully and making substitutions. These are not nutritionally-directed suggestions: I did not take into consideration vitamins, protein counts, or such things as additives, preservatives, or any other health factors.

From the above, you can see that you need not deny your child his or her favorite cakes, cookies, or other treats, just because of a diet. For the weight-reducing program to succeed, the child must not feel deprived. It should, if possible, be an adventure for both of you. It is even possible for it to be fun. There is no reason for any dieter to have only tasteless, watery food. I am in no way suggesting that your child go without the usual "fun foods." I am saying that you can, with a little research and effort, find satisfactory substitutes for high-calorie foods, thus enabling your child to lose weight and still enjoy a range of tastes as well.

It is up to you to investigate what is available in your supermarket and then make the proper choices.

CHAPTER 9
Habits Are
Difficult To Break

We could wipe out childhood obesity in the United States. Prevention is clearly our best weapon. Polio had Dr. Salk; rabies, Dr. Pasteur. You, the parent, can provide the best immunization for the prevention of obesity in your child. Should he or she already be overweight, you hold the best tools for treatment.

I am not a spiritual mentor. I am educated in the field of nutrition and experienced in the physical and emotional treatment of obesity and other eating disorders. I have dealt with the body, the purely physical. I have also delved into only a few of the emotional and psychological elements that are part of the total picture: a) developmental (causes); b) personal, emotional, and social disturbances which obesity sustains; and c) the challenges to life-style and identity which come from treatment and recovery.

It is my sincere hope that my practical advice will be of help to you. The few suggestions I have made are simply a beginning, meant to serve as a springboard for your own research into what is appropriate for your troubled child. I trust you will take what I offer only as suggestions, for, as I have said, every individual is different.

Obesity is not a simple matter. It is extremely complicated, and recovery can be a delicate process. Please turn to your physician, school personnel, and other professionals for physical and psychological aid. We must not neglect the spirit. Your religious counselor is your guide in this matter. For matters of the body, we can turn to our small knowledge: for matters of the spirit, we must turn to God.

Carl Sandburg wrote this rather poignant saying:

"Life is like an onion; you peel off one layer at a time, and sometimes you weep."

Whether shedding a layer of fat or discarding a long-term habit, the difficulties are many. There is pain, and sometimes you weep.

At all times, keep your arms open to receive your child's pain. Hurt can sometimes seem unbearable; the best response in the world is a parent's love. Be your child six or sixteen, the complexities of a weight-loss program can be dealt with. Try to keep the diet as simple as possible. Surround your child with a strong but flexible structure. There must always be room for movement: there are no absolutes.

Sunshine follows rain—hardships, growing pains, emotional and physical hunger pangs, are all part of life. Do not forget to rejoice. God did not mean us to suffer. One of the most tragic things about human nature is that all of us tend to avoid facing reality, and to dream instead of some magical rose garden over that ever-elusive horizon. We forget to enjoy the flowers which are blooming right now in our lives. Taking time to smell the flowers has carried many a child (and many an adult) through stormy weather, through the rain, and into the light of the sun.

Parents, be kind to yourselves. It is an old saying that we can only give what we already have. Expect to make mistakes; forgive yourself immediately; and be honest with yourself and with your child. Admitting your own weaknesses while remaining open will encourage your child to grow in the same way. A weight-loss program can be a means of strengthening your relationship with your child and with your God.

It is always with a smile that I remember one of my patients coming in with a button on her blouse which read: "Please hug me, don't feed me. I am so hungry to be loved."

May your journey with your child be a loving, healthy, and safe one. Should it be rough at times, may you find spiritual soothing and hope to carry on.

Thank you for your time. Your child also thanks you.

Suggestions
for Further Reading

Ashley, Richard and Duggal, Heidi. *Dictionary of Nutrition*. New York: Simon and Schuster, 1976.

Bonow, Raysa Rose. *How to Be a Thin Person*. New York: Random House, 1977.

Kraus, Barbara. *Calories and Carbohydrates*. Third edition. New York: New American Library, 1979.

Maynard, Leslie-Jane. *The Freedom Diet— Games Dieters Play*. New York: Dieters Counseling Service, 1977.

Nidetch, Jean. *The Story of Weight Watchers*. Revised edition. New York: New American Library, 1979.

U.S. Department of Agriculture. *Composition of Foods*. Washington: U.S. Government Printing Office, 1976.